# *A Journey To Home*

## A Preemie Baby Book and NICU Companion Journal

Writing & Design :. Jessica Williams

Artwork & Illustrations :. Lara Payton

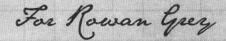

*For Rowan Grey*

Grateful acknowledgement is made to Lara Payton of Dusty Bear Designs for her generosity and creativity in the use of her artwork and illustrations.

Third Edition :. November, 2010

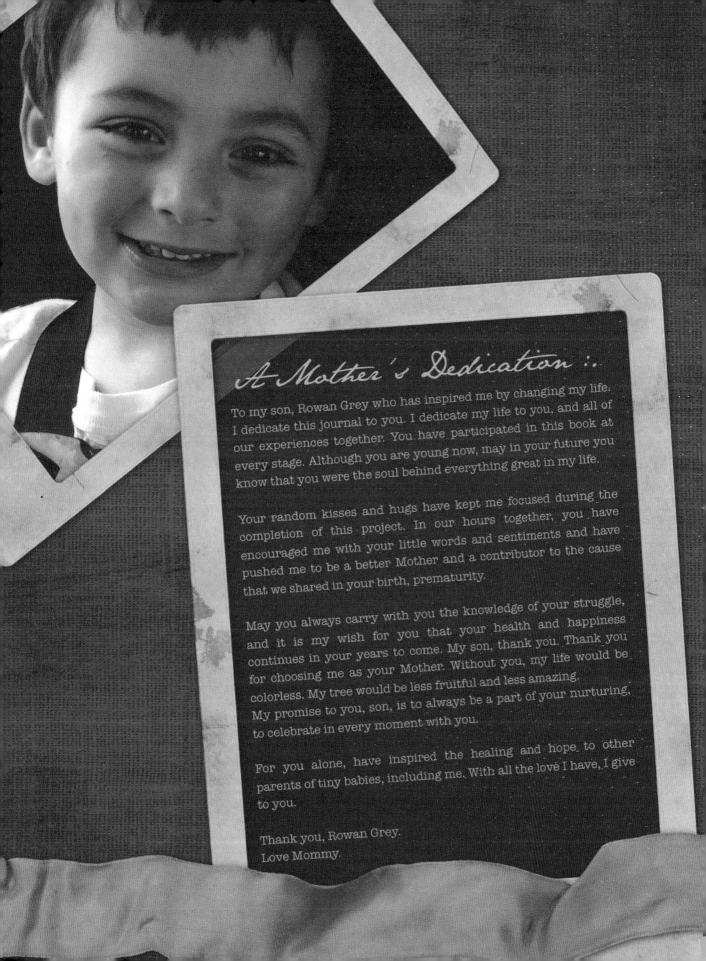

## A Mother's Dedication :..

To my son, Rowan Grey who has inspired me by changing my life.
I dedicate this journal to you. I dedicate my life to you, and all of
our experiences together. You have participated in this book at
every stage. Although you are young now, may in your future you
know that you were the soul behind everything great in my life.

Your random kisses and hugs have kept me focused during the
completion of this project. In our hours together, you have
encouraged me with your little words and sentiments and have
pushed me to be a better Mother and a contributor to the cause
that we shared in your birth, prematurity.

May you always carry with you the knowledge of your struggle,
and it is my wish for you that your health and happiness
continues in your years to come. My son, thank you. Thank you
for choosing me as your Mother. Without you, my life would be
colorless. My tree would be less fruitful and less amazing.
My promise to you, son, is to always be a part of your nurturing,
to celebrate in every moment with you.

For you alone, have inspired the healing and hope to other
parents of tiny babies, including me. With all the love I have, I give
to you.

Thank you, Rowan Grey.
Love Mommy.

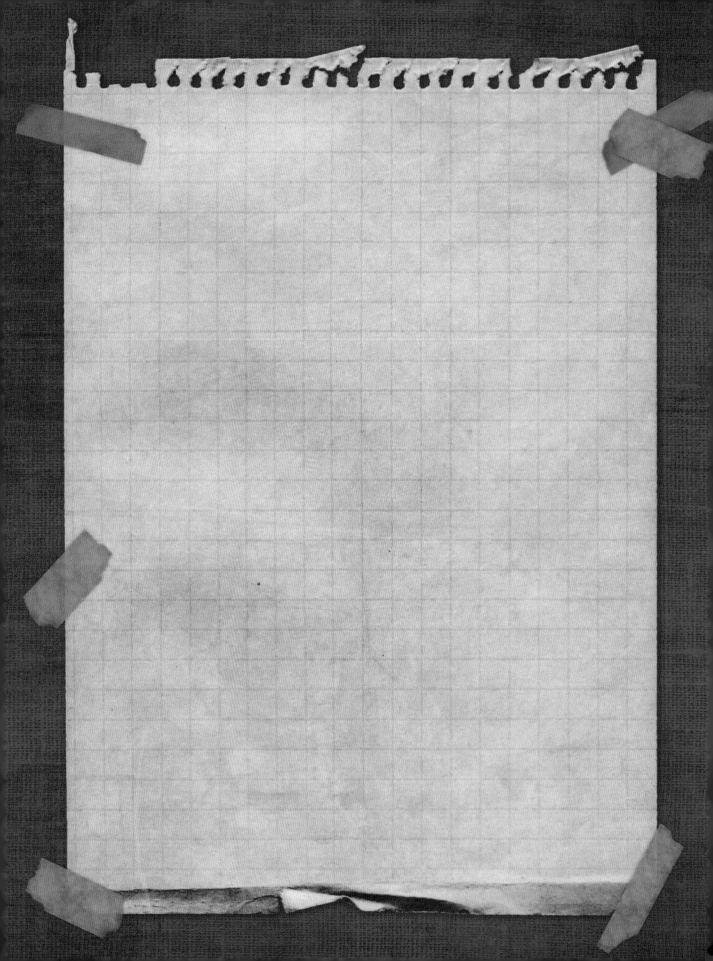

# expecting you

**1**

*Expecting You*
- My Wish for You
- The Day You Came Into My Life
- First Photos of You
- A Letter to My Baby
- Photo Page
- Ten Tiny Fingers, Ten Tiny Toes
- Family Tree
- About Our Family

# Contents.

*Transitioning to Home*

**37**

- Going Home Goals
- Going Home Checklist
- Photo & Journaling Pages
- Contacts & Phone Numbers
- Sentiments
- Going Home
- Baby & Family Care Givers
- Photo & Journaling Pages

# transitioning to home

*Our Home for Awhile*

**13**

- Important Contacts
- Conversion Charts
- Monthly Calendars
- NICU Dictionary
- Milestones & Photos
- My NICU Friends
- Our Firsts
- Moments We Have Shared
- Holidays and Celebrations
- Thoughtful Gifts & Expressions
- NICU Visitors

# our home for awhile

# resources for us

*Resources for Us*

**53**

- Miracle Bebe
- Free Products, Services, Resources & More
- The Story of Rowan Grey
- The Preemie, Devoted to Healing
- The Preemie, Free Downloads
- Preemie Advocacy & Resources

I have expected you for some time now.

We have grown together in anticipation for the day we are able to gaze into each other's eyes for moments that turn into days.

My love for you has healed my heart. Your love for me has made me believe. You are my angel and I am yours. We are miracles to each other; and forever we will grow with strength and love.

I have expected you for some time now.

We have faith that we will be together always. You are a part of me, and I am a part of you. We share one heart and will share our lives for eternity. And for eternity, I will believe that I was meant to be yours. Forever, I will know you have a destiny in my world.

I have expected you for some time now.

We have loved for moments in time that stood still in my heart. Your little body has brought a big soul from heaven. The day you came to me was the day you changed my life forever.

*Expecting You...*

I made a wish, and you came true.

date:

date:_____
_____
_____
_____
_____
_____
_____
_____
_____
_____
_____
_____
_____
_____
_____
_____
_____
_____
_____
_____

# The Day You Came Into My Life.

_____

You were born on _____

at _____ o'clock _____ .

In the city of _____ ,

in the state of _____ .

Your Gestational Age

_____ weeks , _____ days

Height :. _____ _____

Weight :. _____ _____

Baby's Doctor :. _____

First Photos Of You.

A Letter To My Baby...

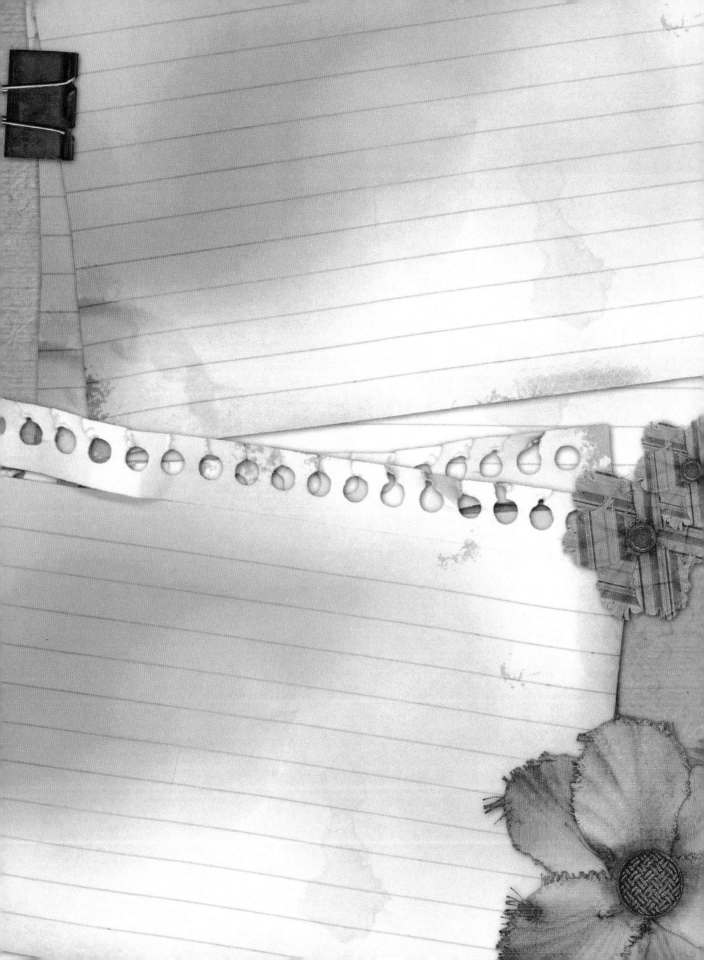

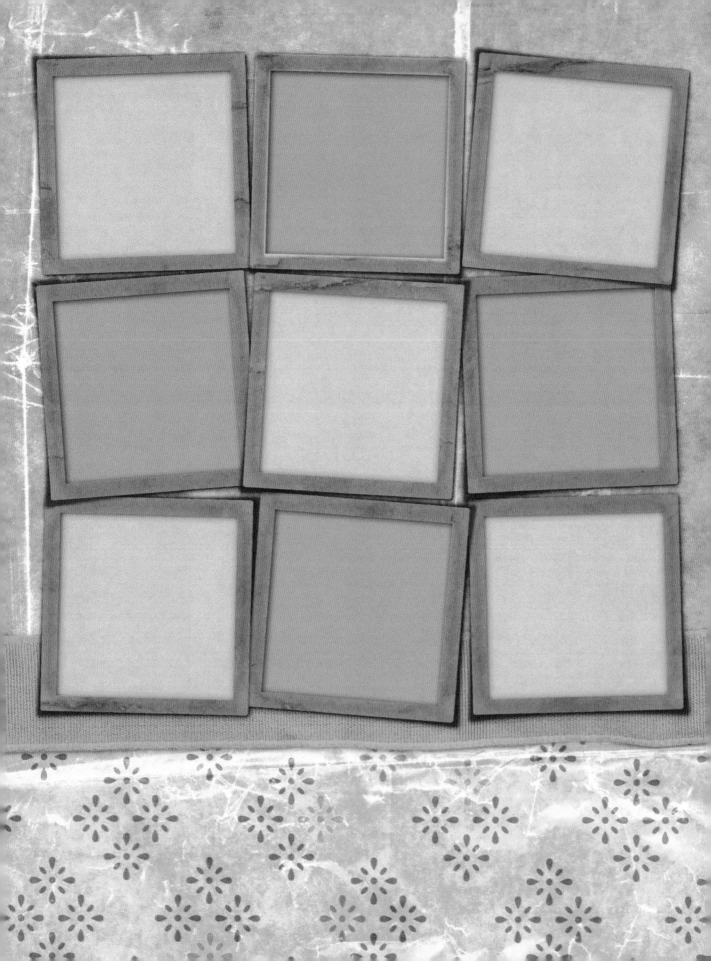

ten tiny fingers

ten tiny toes

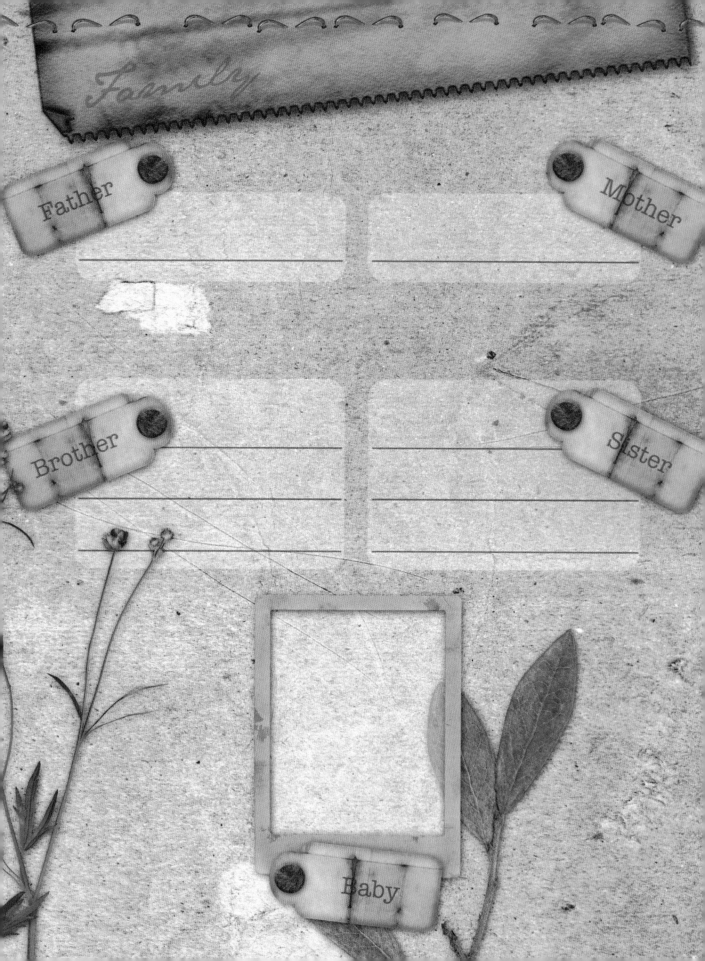

*Family*

Father

Mother

Brother

Sister

Baby

# About Our Family

In my heart I wanted to take you home today, to a place of love, for an infinite stay. For a time your home will be here, in a place not far from me. My dear, my little one, this is your home for awhile.

May your breaths be taken with strength and your tears never be.

In a time our lives will be filled with each other day and night. In a while we will be complete again, just like we used to be.

My wish for you is to see the days fly by with triumphs and growth, then let the time slow the days when we bring you home. Let us be whole in your time of healing. Let us be comforted in our feelings. My love for you is filled with yearning, for dear baby, my heart is hurting.

Make your home for awhile a place of peace, and I will bring you all of the rest. All of the love you should need, all of the moments so tender, I will share with you my heart forever.

*Our Home for Awhile...*

## NICU Receptionist

Contact :. _____

Phone :. _____

## NICU Nurses Line

Contact :. _____

Phone :. _____

## NICU Direct Line to Room

Phone :. _____

## Hospital Receptionist

Phone :. _____

## Emergency Contact

Contact :. _____

Phone :. _____

## OB-GYN

Contact :. _____

Phone :. _____

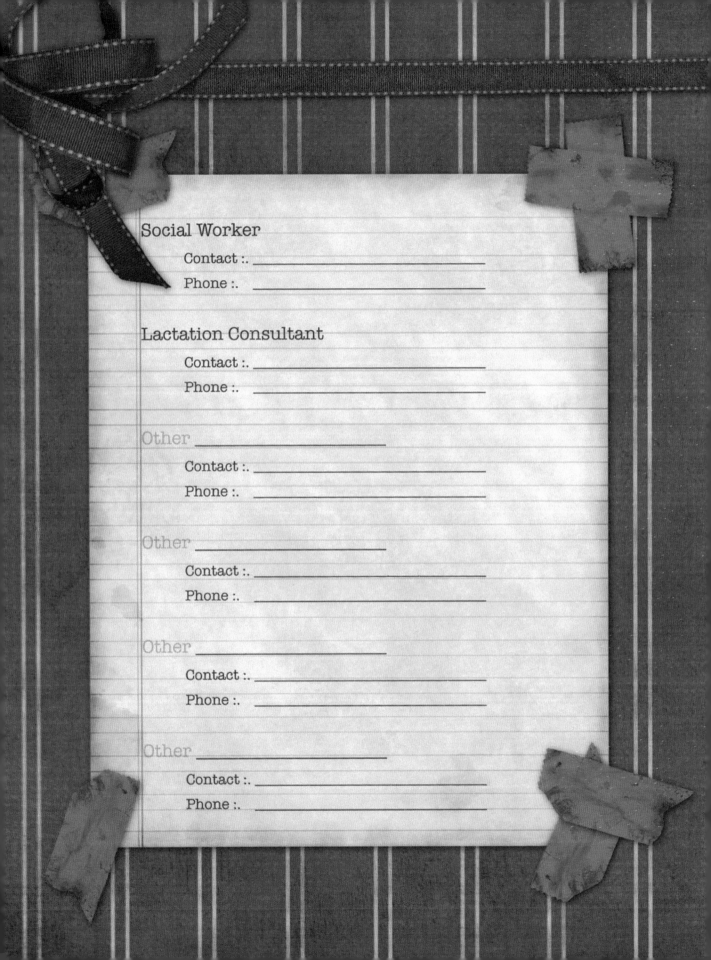

## Social Worker

Contact :. _____

Phone :. _____

## Lactation Consultant

Contact :. _____

Phone :. _____

## Other _____

Contact :. _____

Phone :. _____

## Other _____

Contact :. _____

Phone :. _____

## Other _____

Contact :. _____

Phone :. _____

## Other _____

Contact :. _____

Phone :. _____

# Pounds to Grams Conversion Chart

| | 0 oz | 1 oz | 2 oz | 3 oz | 4 oz | 5 oz | 6 oz | 7 oz | 8 oz | 9 oz | 10 oz | 11 oz | 12 oz | 13 oz | 14 oz | 15 oz |
|---|---|---|---|---|---|---|---|---|---|---|---|---|---|---|---|---|
| **0 lb** | 0 | 28 | 57 | 85 | 113 | 142 | 170 | 198 | 227 | 255 | 283 | 312 | 340 | 369 | 397 | 425 |
| **1 lb** | 453 | 481 | 510 | 534 | 566 | 595 | 623 | 651 | 680 | 708 | 737 | 765 | 793 | 822 | 850 | 878 |
| **2 lbs** | 907 | 936 | 964 | 992 | 1021 | 1049 | 1077 | 1106 | 1134 | 1162 | 1191 | 1219 | 1247 | 1276 | 1304 | 1332 |
| **3 lbs** | 1361 | 1389 | 1417 | 1446 | 1474 | 1503 | 1531 | 1559 | 1588 | 1616 | 1644 | 1673 | 1701 | 1729 | 1758 | 1786 |
| **4 lbs** | 1814 | 1843 | 1871 | 1899 | 1928 | 1956 | 1984 | 2013 | 2041 | 2070 | 2098 | 2126 | 2155 | 2183 | 2211 | 2240 |
| **5 lbs** | 2268 | 2296 | 2325 | 2353 | 2381 | 2410 | 2438 | 2466 | 2495 | 2523 | 2551 | 2580 | 2608 | 2637 | 2665 | 2693 |
| **6 lbs** | 2722 | 2750 | 2778 | 2807 | 2835 | 2863 | 2892 | 2920 | 2948 | 2977 | 3005 | 3033 | 3062 | 3090 | 3118 | 3147 |
| **7 lbs** | 3175 | 3203 | 3232 | 3260 | 3289 | 3317 | 3345 | 3374 | 3402 | 3430 | 3459 | 3487 | 3515 | 3544 | 3572 | 3600 |
| **8 lbs** | 3629 | 3657 | 3685 | 3714 | 3742 | 3770 | 3799 | 3827 | 3856 | 3884 | 3912 | 3941 | 3969 | 3997 | 4026 | 4054 |

## Metric Conversion Chart

| | |
|---|---|
| 1 pound (lb.) | 453 grams |
| 1 pound (lb.) | .453 kilograms |
| 1 pound (lb.) | 16 ounces |
| 1 inch | 2.54 centimeters |
| 1 ounce | 29.6 cc (30 cc) |
| 98.6° | 37c |

## Other Conversions

| Unit | Unit |
|---|---|
| | |
| | |

## Head Circumference

| Date | Circumference |
| --- | --- |
|  |  |
|  |  |
|  |  |
|  |  |

## Height Chart

| Date | Height |
| --- | --- |
|  |  |
|  |  |
|  |  |
|  |  |
|  |  |
|  |  |

## Weight Chart

| Date | Weight |
| --- | --- |
|  |  |
|  |  |
|  |  |
|  |  |
|  |  |
|  |  |

| Sunday | Monday | Tuesday | Wednesday | Thursday | Friday | Saturday |
|--------|--------|---------|-----------|----------|--------|----------|
|        |        |         |           |          |        |          |
|        |        |         |           |          |        |          |
|        |        |         |           |          |        |          |
|        |        |         |           |          |        |          |
|        |        |         |           |          |        |          |

## Monthly Events & Reminders

| Date | Event or Reminder | Date | Event or Reminder |
|------|-------------------|------|-------------------|
|      |                   |      |                   |
|      |                   |      |                   |
|      |                   |      |                   |
|      |                   |      |                   |
|      |                   |      |                   |
|      |                   |      |                   |
|      |                   |      |                   |
|      |                   |      |                   |

| Sunday | Monday | Tuesday | Wednesday | Thursday | Friday | Saturday |
|--------|--------|---------|-----------|----------|--------|----------|
|        |        |         |           |          |        |          |
|        |        |         |           |          |        |          |
|        |        |         |           |          |        |          |
|        |        |         |           |          |        |          |
|        |        |         |           |          |        |          |

# Monthly Events & Reminders

| Date | Event or Reminder | Date | Event or Reminder |
|------|-------------------|------|-------------------|
|      |                   |      |                   |
|      |                   |      |                   |
|      |                   |      |                   |
|      |                   |      |                   |
|      |                   |      |                   |
|      |                   |      |                   |
|      |                   |      |                   |
|      |                   |      |                   |

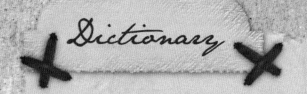
# Dictionary

## apnea of prematurity
Temporary cessation of breathing. Premature babies will often "forget" to breathe until they grow out of their prematurity.

## aspiration
Inhalation of material (formula, meconium or stomach juice) into the trachea (windpipe) and lungs.

## bilirubin
A pigment produced in the breakdown of red blood cells that appears as yellow skin coloring (jaundice).

## bililights
Lights placed over or under the infant to help in the breakdown of bilirubin, thereby reducing jaundice.

## blood gases
Laboratory test to determine the amount of oxygen and carbon dioxide in the blood.

## bradycardia
Slow heart rate.

## cat scan
A special X-ray study which uses a computer to create an image of the body or a part of the body.

## cc's
Cubic centimeters. 30 cc's = 1 fluid ounce.

## chest p.t.
Vibration on the chest to loosen secretions and suctioning to remove mucous from the lungs.

## cpap (continuous positive airway pressure)
A device that reminds baby to breathe by forcing air in the nose.

## cyanosis
Condition in which the skin, lips and nails are blue from lack of oxygen in the blood.

## eeg (electroencephalogram)
Test done to measure brain wave pattern or to look for seizures.

## echo (echocardiogram)
A heart test done with sound waves to pick up the image of the heart and its vessels through the chest wall without hurting the baby.

## gavage feeding
A tube is placed through the baby's nose or in its mouth, down its throat to its stomach. Breast milk or formula can be given to the baby through the tube.

## gestational age
Age of the baby in weeks, determined from the time of conception.

## hyalin membrane disease (rds)
A respiratory disease often seen in premature infants caused by immature lung development.

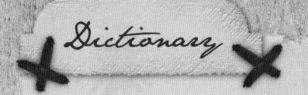

# Dictionary

**hyperalimentation**
Giving nutrients through a vein for babies who cannot be fed by mouth.

**incubator** (isolette)
Enclosed beds for the babies that are temperature controlled for babies who cannot maintain or regulate their own temperatures.

**intravenous** (iv)
Introduction of fluids into a vein.

**intubation**
Insertion of a tube through the nose or mouth into the trachea (windpipe).

**i & o** (intake and output)
Total amount of fluid taken in, then lost as urine, stool or perspiration.

**jaundice**
Yellowish color of the skin caused by the buildup of bilirubin.

**kangaroo care**
Holding a baby against one's chest, so there is skin-to-skin contact.

**meconium**
A baby's first stool, which is greenish or black.

**nasal cannula**
A special tubing that is used to give oxygen through the nose, making holding and feeding easier.

**npo**
Baby will get nothing to eat by mouth.

**picc** (pick line)
A special IV line used to provide fluids into a vein. In general, a PICC line is very stable and lasts longer than a typical IV. Also known as PCVC.

**pneumothorax**
Accumulation of air between the outer lining of the lung and the chest wall, causing collapse of the lung.

**respirator** (ventilator)
A machine that breathes for an infant. Also referred to as a vent.

**rounds**
The gathering of doctors, nurses and other health care professionals to discuss the condition and care of patients.

**sepsis**
Infection.

**spinal tap** (lp)
Insertion of a small needle through the back into the spinal column to obtain a sample of spinal fluid.

**umbilical catheter**
(umbilical line)
A tiny plastic tube inserted into the blood vessel of a baby's umbilical cord used to give the baby fluids and to withdraw blood samples.

**vital signs**
Temperature, heart rate, respiration.

Date :. _____ Milestone :. _____
Notes :. 
_____
_____
_____

Date :. _____ Milestone :. _____
Notes :. 
_____
_____
_____

Date :. _____ Milestone :. _____
Notes :. 
_____
_____
_____

Date :. _____ Milestone :. _____
Notes :. 
_____
_____
_____

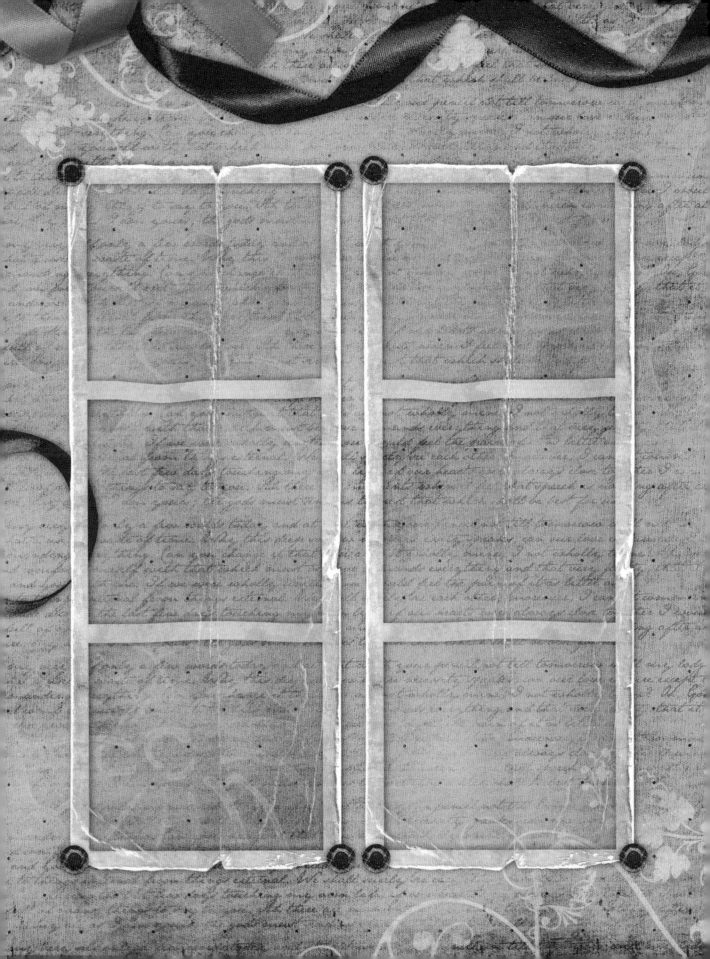

Date :. _____ Milestone :. _____
Notes :.
_____
_____
_____

Date :. _____ Milestone :. _____
Notes :.
_____
_____
_____

Date :. _____ Milestone :. _____
Notes :.
_____
_____
_____

Date :. _____ Milestone :. _____
Notes :.
_____
_____
_____

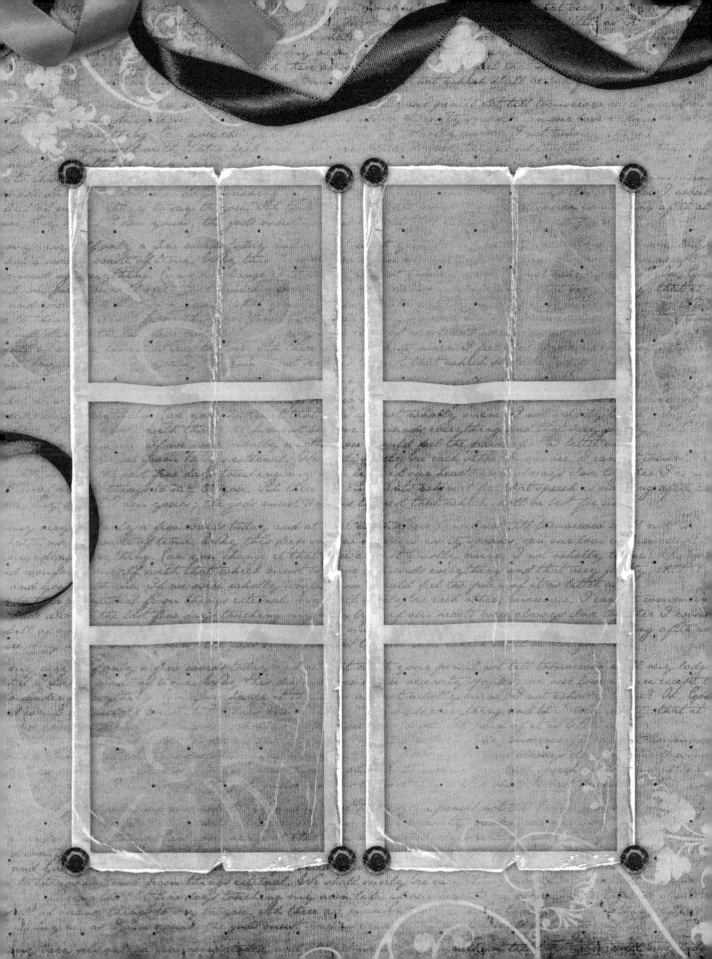

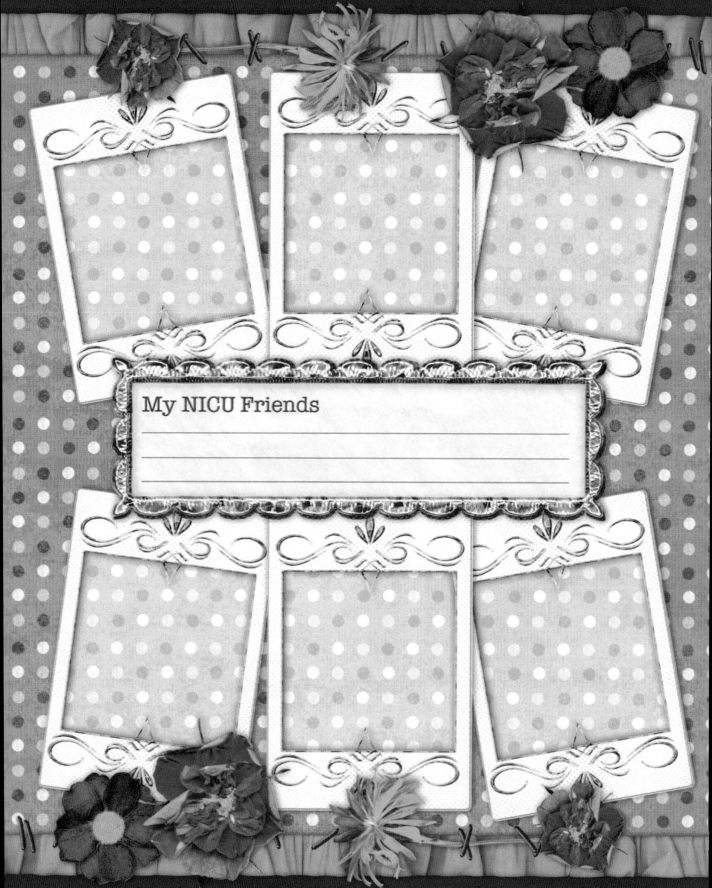

My NICU Friends

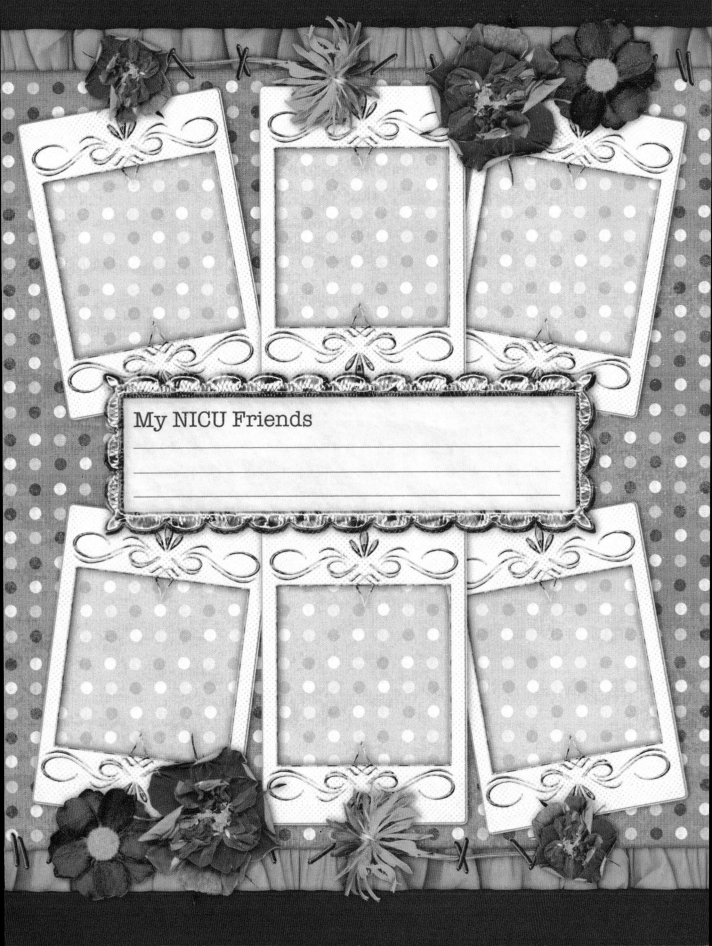

My NICU Friends

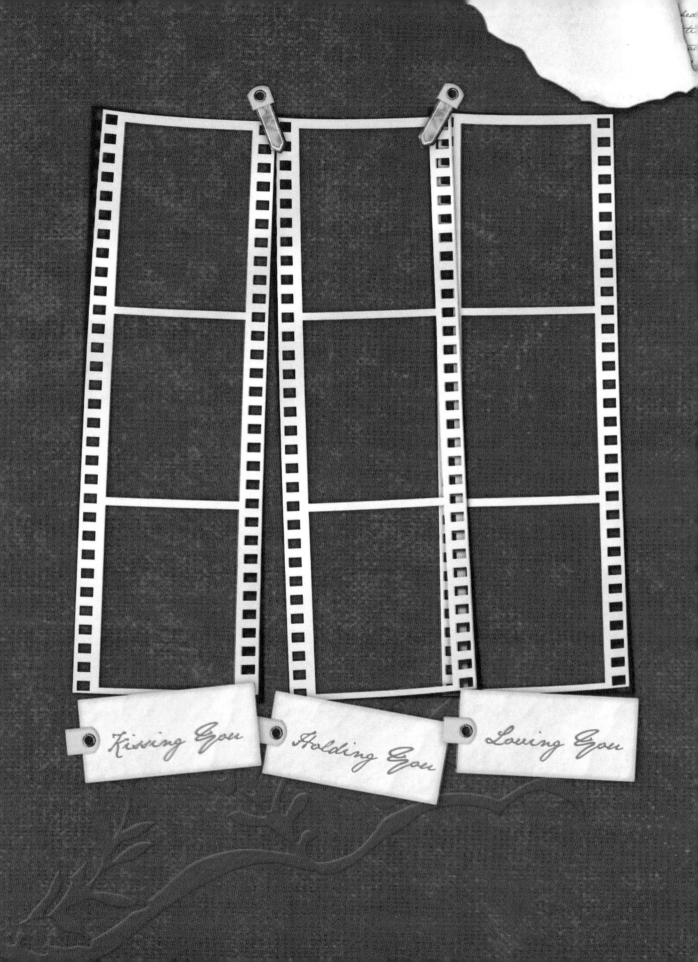

Kissing You    Holding You    Loving You

my heart ached

first time, I felt whole. When I
...d you for the fi...
las...

Our first touch was

Our first kiss was

Our first hold was

Moments We Have Shared

Holidays and Celebrations

Holidays and Celebrations

TO DARLING BABY

Date:: ___/___/___     From:: _____

Gift:: _____

_____ Thank You Sent:: ___

Date:: ___/___/___     From:: _____

Gift:: _____

_____ Thank You Sent:: ___

Date:: ___/___/___     From:: _____

Gift:: _____

_____ Thank You Sent:: ___

Date:: ___/___/___     From:: _____

Gift:: _____

_____ Thank You Sent:: ___

Date:: ___/___/___     From:: _____

Gift:: _____

_____ Thank You Sent:: ___

Date:: ___/___/___     From:: _____

Gift:: _____

_____ Thank You Sent:: ___

Date:: ___/___/___     From:: _____     Thank You Sent:: _____

Gift:: _____

Date:: ___/___/___     From:: _____     Thank You Sent:: _____

Gift:: _____

Date:: ___/___/___     From:: _____     Thank You Sent:: _____

Gift:: _____

Date:: ___/___/___     From:: _____     Thank You Sent:: _____

Gift:: _____

Date:: ___/___/___     From:: _____     Thank You Sent:: _____

Gift:: _____

Date:: ___/___/___     From:: _____     Thank You Sent:: _____

Gift:: _____

Date:: ___/___/___     From:: _____     Thank You Sent:: _____

Gift:: _____

# NICU Visitors

Date :. _____          Visitor :. _____

Sentiments :.

_____

_____

_____


Date :. _____          Visitor :. _____

Sentiments :.

_____

_____

_____


Date :. _____          Visitor :. _____

Sentiments :.

_____

_____

_____

# NICU Visitors

Date :. _____          Visitor :. _____

Sentiments :.

_____

_____

_____


Date :. _____          Visitor :. _____

Sentiments :.

_____

_____

_____


Date :. _____          Visitor :. _____

Sentiments :.

_____

_____

_____

The thought of you in my arms forever, the thought of you and I together... In a place far from here there is a world that we will share your happy coos and little smiles. I will delight in our moments and treasure our worlds as one.

The thought of you in my life fills me with a sense of wonder. How our souls met and how infinite our love is for each other.

This place we will share will be a place of peace, a universe of happiness, and arms full of tenderness.

My child, my promise to you is forever.

Let us go home now and share the moments we have missed. Let us walk in the days ahead far from the thoughts of sorrow. Let us travel in our world with strength, faith and wellness, for my prayers are for your tomorrows.

Transitioning to Home...

# I'm Gaining Weight

Date :. _____ / _____ / _____          Weight :. _____

Notes :. _____

Date :. _____ / _____ / _____          Weight :. _____

Notes :. _____

Date :. _____ / _____ / _____          Weight :. _____

Notes :. _____

Date :. _____ / _____ / _____          Weight :. _____

Notes :. _____

# I'm Taking Feeds

Date :. _____ / _____ / _____

_____ ____ ____ ____ ____ ____ ____ ____ _____

Date :. _____ / _____ / _____

_____ ____ ____ ____ ____ ____ ____ ____ _____

Date :. _____ / _____ / _____

_____ ____ ____ ____ ____ ____ ____ ____ _____

Date :. _____ / _____ / _____

_____ ____ ____ ____ ____ ____ ____ ____ _____

# I'm Holding My Temperature

Date :. _____/_____/_____     Temp :. _____

Notes :. _____

Date :. _____/_____/_____     Temp :. _____

Notes :. _____

Date :. _____/_____/_____     Temp :. _____

Notes :. _____

Date :. _____/_____/_____     Temp :. _____

Notes :. _____

# Other Episodes

Date :. ____/____/____          Bradycardia/Apnea/Other

Notes :. _____

Date :. ____/____/____          Bradycardia/Apnea/Other

Notes :. _____

Date :. ____/____/____          Bradycardia/Apnea/Other

Notes :. _____

Date :. ____/____/____          Bradycardia/Apnea/Other

Notes : _____

# going home checklist

CPR training

date:. _____

Eye Exam

date:. _____

Apnea monitor training

date:. _____

Hearing Exam

date:. _____

Circumcision

date:. _____

Preemie Developmental Evaluation

date:. _____

Hep B vaccination

date:. _____

_____

date:. _____

# going home checklist

_____

date:. _____

_____

date:. _____

_____

date:. _____

_____

date:. _____

_____

date:. _____

_____

date:. _____

_____

date:. _____

_____

date:. _____

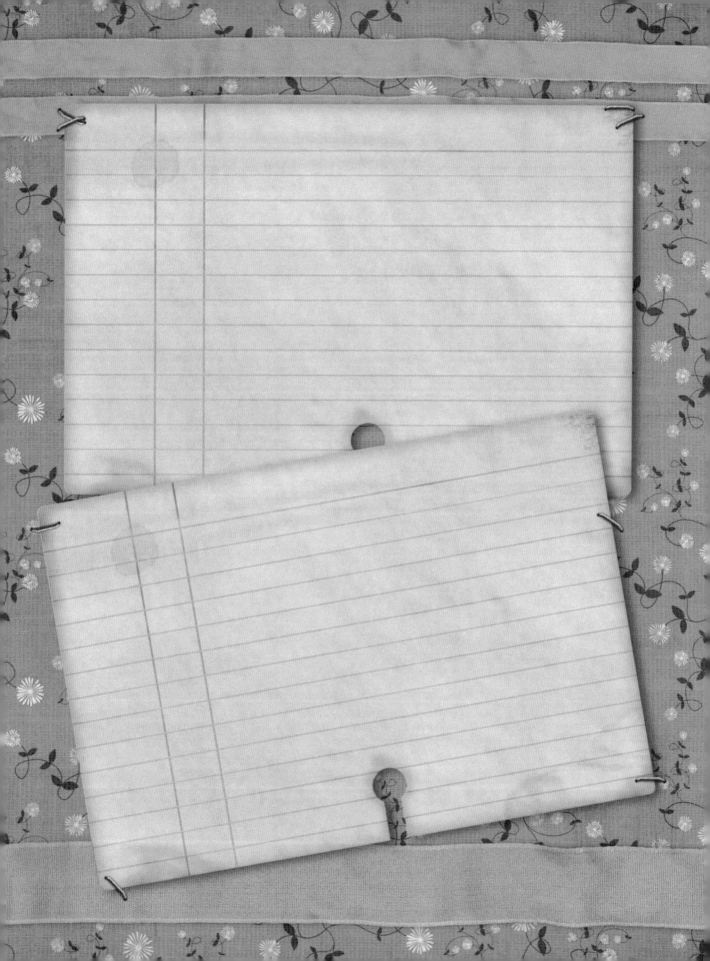

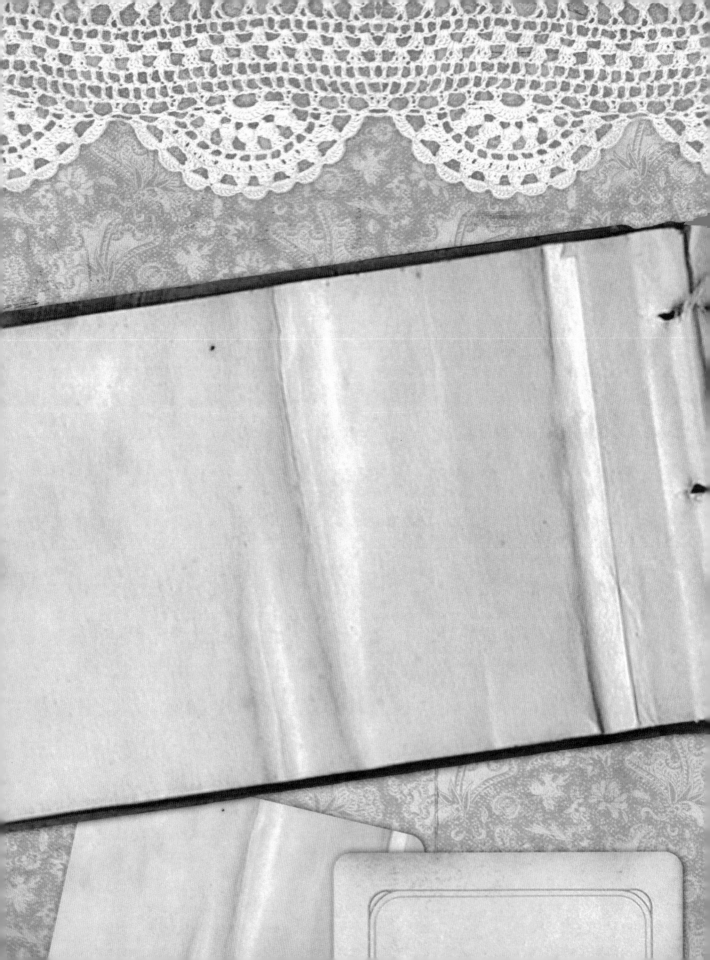

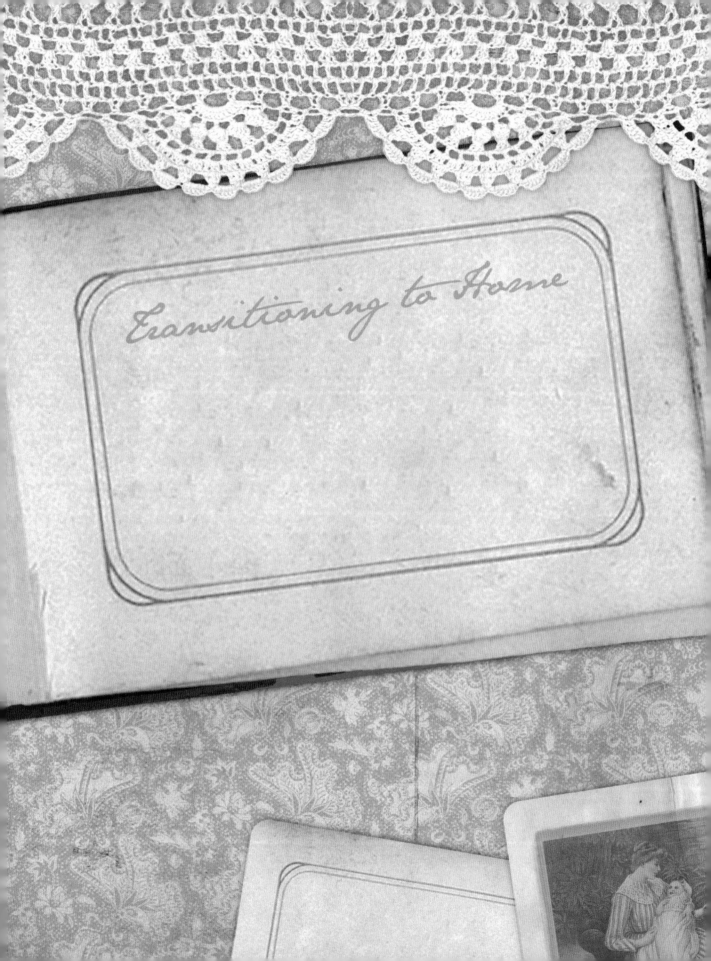

Transitioning to Home

NICU :.

Phone Number :.

Baby's Pediatrician :.

Phone Number :.

Family Physician :.

Phone Number :.

Local Hospital :.

Phone Number :.

Visiting Nurses Line :.

Phone Number :.

Medical Supplies :.

Phone Number :.

Insurance Company :.

Phone Number :.

Other :.

Phone Number :.

Other :.

Phone Number :.

# Sentiments

# Going Home

Date : _____

_____

_____

_____

_____

_____

_____

_____

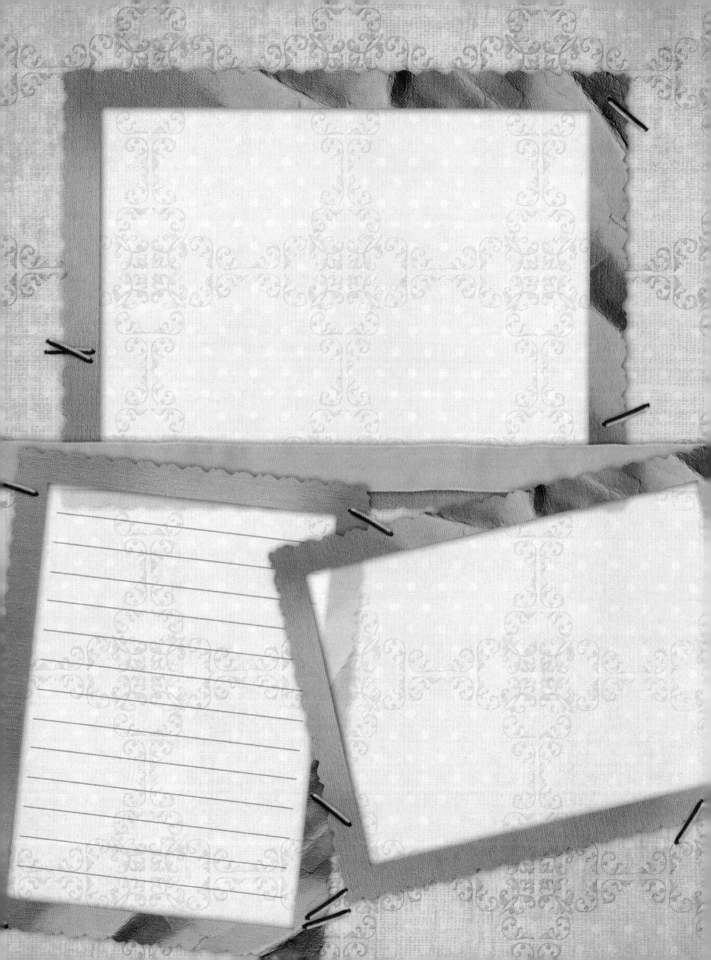

name :. _____

phone :. _____

email :. _____

job :. _____

availability :.

    Sun :. _____    Mon :. _____

    Tue :. _____    Wed :. _____

    Thu :. _____    Frid :. _____

    Sat :. _____    _____

hourly rate :. _____

other :. _____

_____

_____

_____

## Baby & Family Care Givers

name :. _____

phone :. _____

email :. _____

job :. _____

availability :.

    Sun :. _____    Mon :. _____

    Tue :. _____    Wed :. _____

    Thu :. _____    Frid :. _____

    Sat :. _____    _____

hourly rate :. _____

other :. _____

_____

_____

_____

name :. _____

phone :. _____

email :. _____

job :. _____

availability :.

        Sun :. _____      Mon :. _____

        Tue :. _____      Wed :. _____

        Thu :. _____      Frid :. _____

        Sat :. _____      _____

hourly rate :. _____

other :. _____

_____

_____

_____

_____

name :. _____

phone :. _____

email :. _____

job :. _____

availability :.

        Sun :. _____      Mon :. _____

        Tue :. _____      Wed :. _____

        Thu :. _____      Frid :. _____

        Sat :. _____      _____

hourly rate :. _____

other :. _____

_____

_____

_____

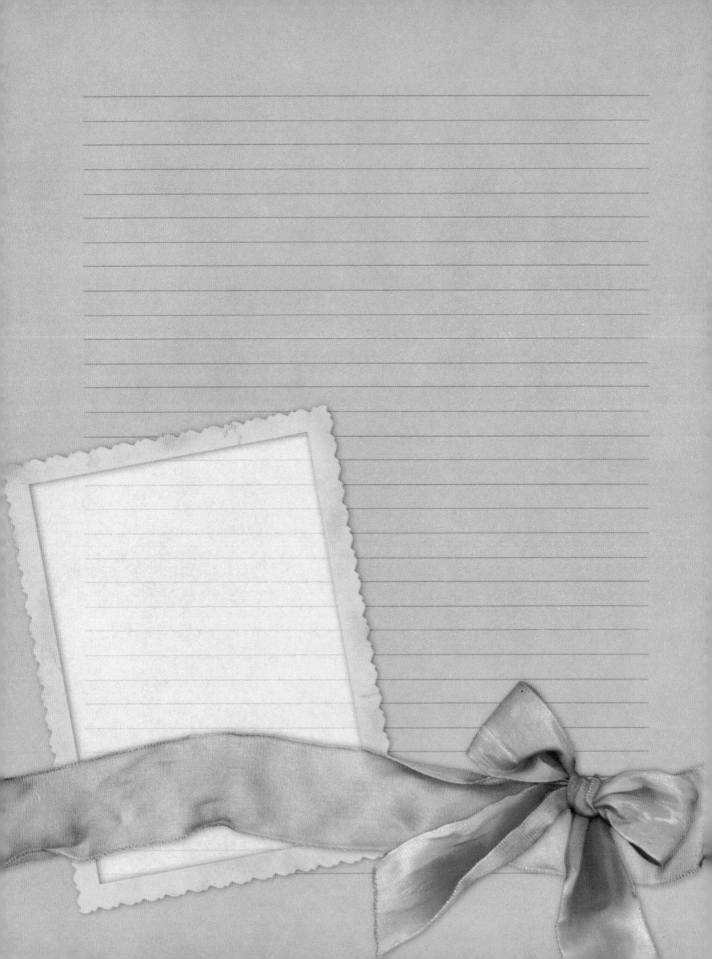

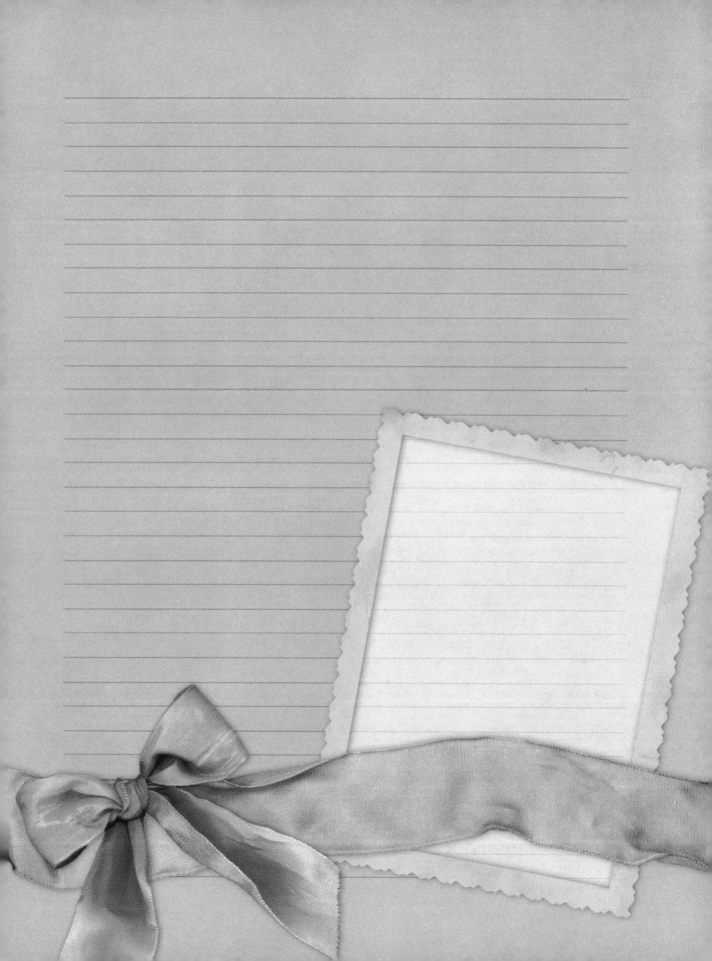

In our time together, we are not alone. For you and I seek healing within ourselves and long for company in our future days.

For us, I will be open with my heart and hold my hand out to others in need. For I am a part of the healing of others and ourselves. My love, you are my driving inspiration. We are not in a secluded battle and your smiles bring me the ambition to reach out.

I am your advocate and you are my spirit. I will take the time to learn, grow, foster and care for us. I will find other miracles in their same quest. We are one, and one within a world of others just like us.

My dedication is to you, to your health and healing. My dedication is to my wellness as a parent and our future together. My baby, for us.

Resources for Us...

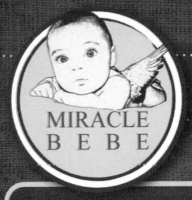

**MIRACLE BEBE**

*from small beginnings come great things.*

Founded in early 2008, Miracle Bebe became an organization dedicated to the awareness of prematurity. With over 500,000 families touched by prematurity in the United States this year, having a preemie is not something a family can predict. That being said, having a premature infant is filled with many surprises.

My hope is to provide knowledge, support and resources for parents and their child(ren). Miracle Bebe was the outcome of hope for all babies born too soon. "Little did I know what to expect over the next 33 days, let alone the years that followed our NICU stay."

Miracle Bebe offers products, services and resources for families. The site continues to grow, and is maintained with freebies and information. From learning to crochet preemie hats to reading stories about other preemies, families will find a comprehensive resource at miraclebebe.com.

## MiracleBebe.com

:: A Journey To Home,
   A NICU companion

:: Made for a Miracle Preemie
   Baby Bag

:: Baby Announcements for
   Preemies

:: Scrapbooking Pages

:: Volunteerism

:: Learn to Crochet Preemie
   Hats

:: Gift Suggestions

:: Resources

:: Scrapbooking Freebies

:: NICU Dictionary

:: Preemie Clip Art

:: Stories of Preemies,
   share yours

products, services, resources & more.

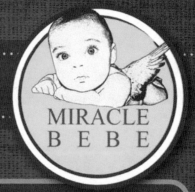

MIRACLE
BEBE

**LARGEST DIGITAL
SCRAPBOOKING SITE FOR**

# Preemies

## www.miraclebebe.com

| digital files | free printable sheets | hybrid scrapbooking options |
| original designs | free isolette reminder cards | & more

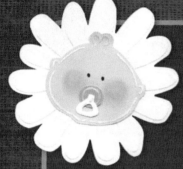

**MANY DESIGNS TO CHOOSE FROM!**

# PREEMIE BABY ANNOUNCEMENTS

Get a customized baby announcement emailed directly to you. Send photo and baby information to info@miraclebebe.com and receive a printable file for your home computer. Limited time offer.

**PRINTING OPTIONS ARE AVAILABLE WITH US :.**
100 announcements, 100 envelopes & free shipping $50.00

## FREE

## Share Your Story

Sharing compassionate stories, challenges, successes and more about prematurity can be extremely healing. Whether writing or reading, our community of parents invite you to share at Miracle Bebe. Come join us and email your story to info@miraclebebe.com

## MADE FOR A MIRACLE

:: Printable Instructions
:: Video Tutorials
:: Sizing Charts
:: and More

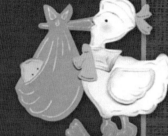

## Learn To Crochet Preemie Hats

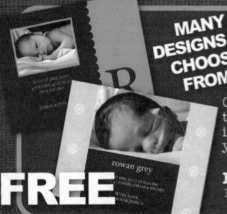

My name is Rowan Grey. I am 4 days old. I was born on a Friday, and I came quite unexpectedly. It wasn't that I was in a hurry meet the world, it was that my mother had a medical condition which doctors could not treat. Despite my early arrival, I came out with loud cries, and kicks. Everyone in the delivery room noticed me right away. Some said I was a handsome boy, and others said I was very tall. Weighing 3 lbs. and 4 oz. my mom was surprised that I was 16.3" in length. (Full term babies are about 19" to 20". I had worked very hard at growing.)

My Dad is Jarrod, he is were I get my good looks and height from. We share almost every trait, except for my personality... That I owe to my mom. My mom is Jessica, and she is an incredibly sensitive and an affectionate lady who loves to hold me.

You will often see her cooing over me, and sometimes shedding tears. She is very happy with me and my progress, but is lonely and would like to bring me home just as soon as she can.

My mom and dad tried to have me for several years, so I am very important to them. They believe that I am their 'miracle' baby, and that I was heaven sent. After I was born, my dad and the kind people at Children's Hospital escorted me to my suite in the Neonatal Intensive Care Unit. That is when Dad named me, Rowan Grey. I knew that my stay would include all the amenities, extreme pampering, and of course, lots of love. It is just the sort of treatment a little man like me needs. I have been here 4 days now, and I have met the nicest nurses and doctors, ever! Dr. John, Dr. Howard and Dr. Dave check in on me often, and order many hugs. My nurses and therapists greet me every day with their big smiles and warm hearts. Some of my favorites are Cole, Mandy, Kelly, Kim (and the other Kim), Lucy, and Wendy. Not to mention all the girls upstairs who took care of me and my mommy before I was born.

Overall, my care was complete with daily visits from my parents, doctors and nurses. I made a couple of trips outside of my room to other areas of the hospital, but my biggest love is the kangaroo care that I so desperately needed from both mom and dad.

After 32 days, my parents were given the opportunity to stay overnight with me in a special room. I had my own bassinet and they complained about the futon. Dad slept a lot while Mom kept her eye on me all night long. To this day, I think she is still catching up on her sleep. I had a couple of quick alarms that were very brief if not even false. The nurses on the outside were only to assist us if we had any emergency of which we had none.

The next day,

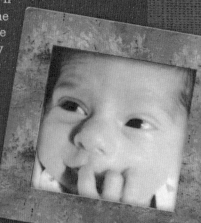

# the story of rowan grey.

was back to my NICU room where we spent hours waiting for evaluations from medical staff and doctors, and then we got the ok. This is me on day 33 leaving the NICU. I was a sleepy baby for many months. We played very little at home. I wore an apnea monitor for three months, it was assuring to my mother that I was breathing well throughout the days and nights. After gaining more and more confidence, and by doctor's orders we were ready to take off the monitor and send it back to the hospital.

I receive normal checkups now, I have outgrown all of my pediatricians expectations and have passed my NICU follow-up with flying colors. I receive my RSV shots on a monthly basis and could possibly continue them next year. I am a lucky little man, I know that, and Mom and Dad know that. We owe a lot of my progress to prayer, medical intervention and just plain hope.

I am over eight months old now, and looking forward to my first birthday and the possibility of eating cake. I am rolling over very well, but remember I am really a five and a half month old little man. If I cannot eat cake this August, Mom says she will have a gestational birthday party for me as well. I just want that cake!

From Mom :.

Rowan is three years now, and looking back at all of the procedures, stages of development, I can only advise other parents to take it one day at a time. The thought of 'what-if' always lingers in the back of your mind, but focus only on right now and what your preemie has to offer you, which is a lot of love.

Prematurity is painful. It takes so much of your heart to go through this in life. Looking at Rowan now, I know that setting my fears aside and going forward with the day made us better preemie parents.

I hope all of you fellow preemies are doing well, we cannot count our blessings enough. Our thoughts and prayers are with you all.

Rowan Grey & Mommy

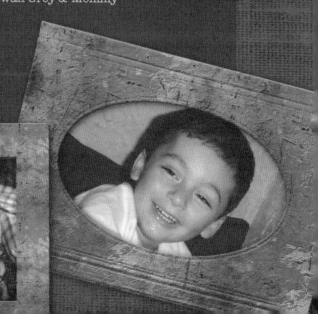

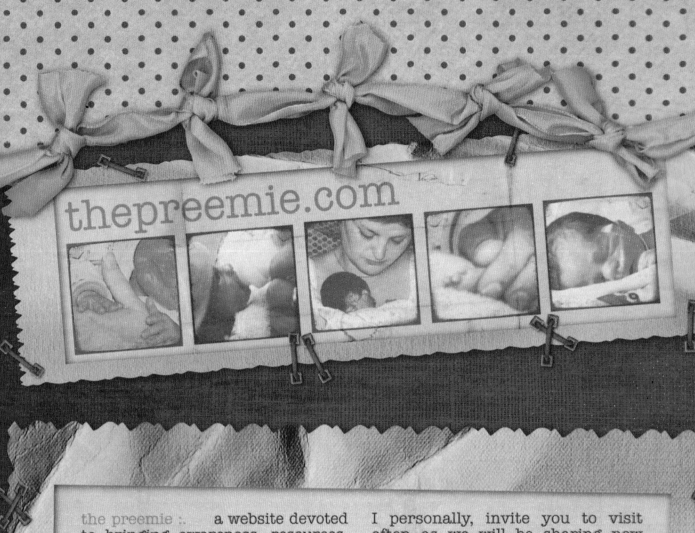

# thepreemie.com

**the preemie :.** a website devoted to bringing awareness, resources, and celebration in the moments of prematurity through healing. a comprehensive resource for all parents and families touched by prematurity. a companion through all nicu experiences.

## follow us :.

for updates, offers, stories and more... search thepreemie on your favorite blog sites.

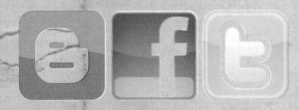

I personally, invite you to visit often as we will be sharing new resources, often. Within these internet pages you will find information regarding a new version of 'A Journey to Home, A Preemie Baby Book and NICU Companion Journal'. In full publication, this diary is a resource for families in the NICU and a preemie baby book full of memory pages. You will also find other organizations that specialize in the healing and hope little babies who find themselves in the hospital for days, sometimes months after birth. The Preemie also offers links to free activities that would be useful for parents spending time in the NICU.

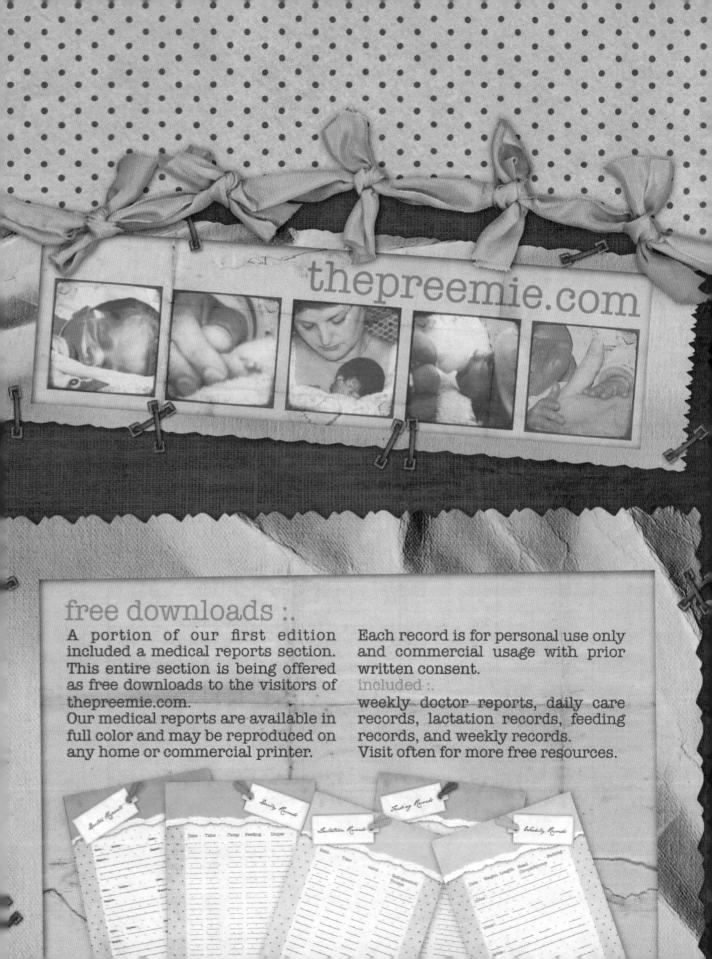

# thepreemie.com

## free downloads :.

A portion of our first edition included a medical reports section. This entire section is being offered as free downloads to the visitors of thepreemie.com.

Our medical reports are available in full color and may be reproduced on any home or commercial printer.

Each record is for personal use only and commercial usage with prior written consent.

included :.

weekly doctor reports, daily care records, lactation records, feeding records, and weekly records.

Visit often for more free resources.

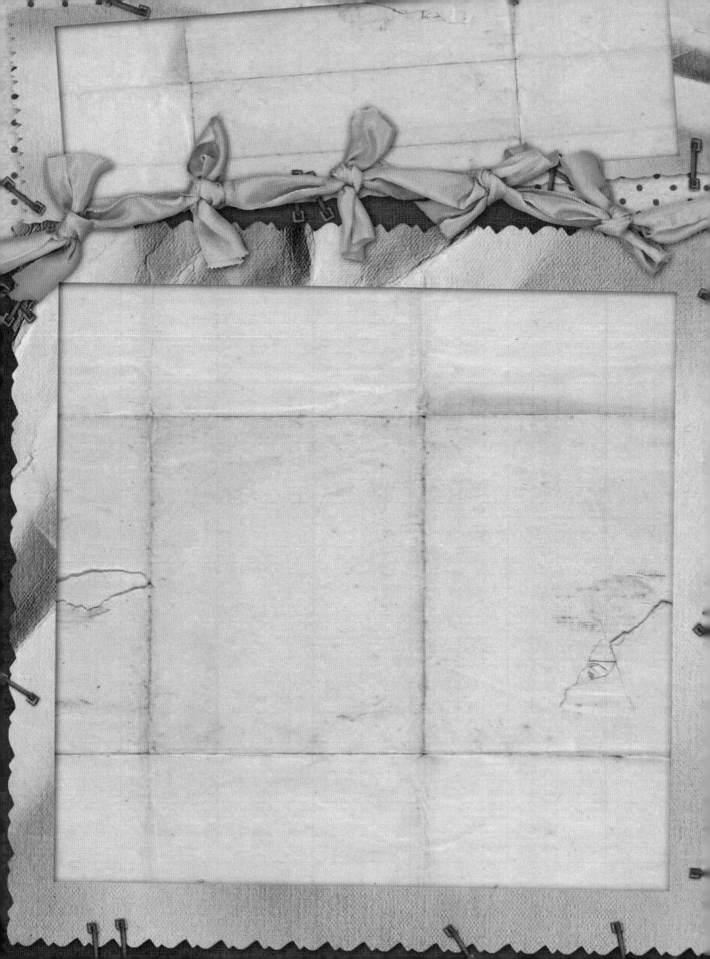

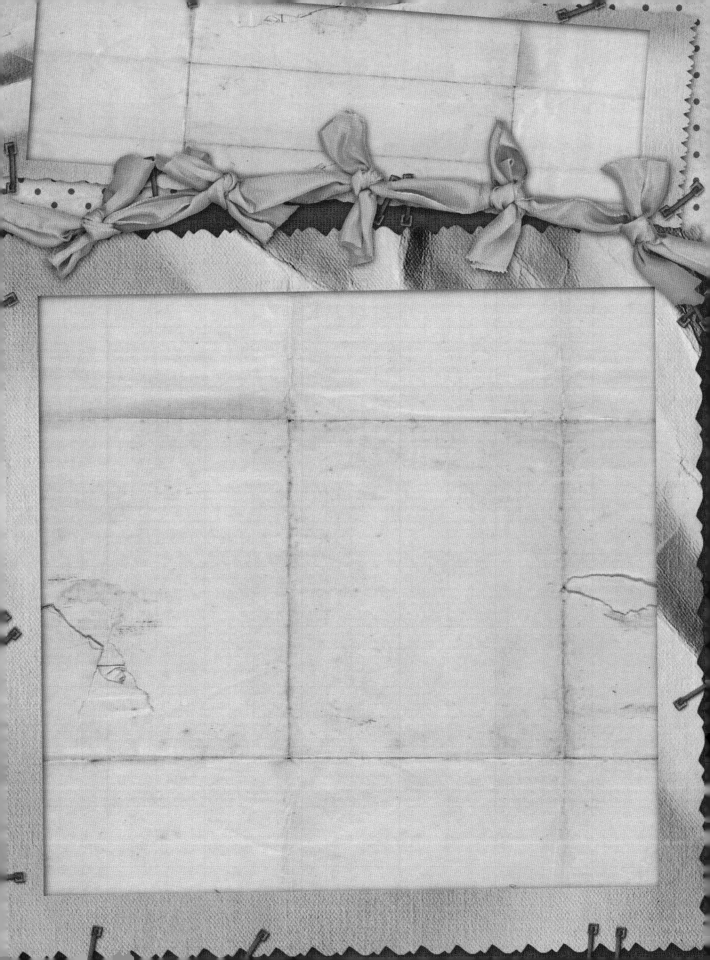

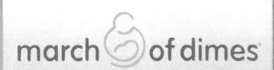

## march of dimes®

**Educate and Advocate**
**Fundraise**
**Volunteer Virtually**
**Time and Talent**

*Share Your Story*

An online community for NICU families.
Participate in online discussions. start a
blog, or just make friends.
Join today :. www.shareyourstory.org

Username :. _____

Password :. _____

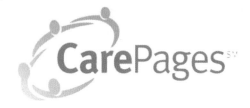

## CarePages℠

Share your story. Build your
Support circle.

CarePages websites are free
patient blogs that connect friends
and family during a health
challenge

Visit: . www.carepages.com

Username :. _____

Password :. _____

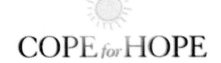

## COPE for HOPE

Promoting the health of children,
teens, and families through stressful times.

**C**reating **O**pportunities for **P**arent
**E**mpowerment with our Evidence-Based
**COPE** Programs™

## COPE NICU Program Information

For parents, please contact us by email at
info@copeforhope.com or by phone at
1-607-664-6159 to find out how you can purchase
their program. Please visit www.copeforhope.com

## PREEMIES TODAY

National Preemie Families Support Network

Preemies Today is a 501(c)(3)
nonprofit organization. Our mission is
to provide outreach and support
programs to families of infants born
prematurely beginning at birth and
throughout childhood. We are located
in the Washington DC metropolitan
area and have local events in
Northern Virginia, Maryland, and DC.

To contact us regarding our programs
email info@preemiestoday.org. Visit
us at www.preemiestoday.org

# Inspire

*together we're better*

*"I am not alone as long as this web site is here for me"*

For more information, visit :. www.inspire.com

## More Resources

_____
_____
_____
_____
_____
_____
_____
_____
_____
_____
_____

All resources listed are provided only as a guide to a variety of online products and services associated with the cause of prematurity in infants and does not imply an endorsement of the information or services provided. This information is not offered to be interpreted as medical or professional advice. Please review all medical information with your Neonatologist, Pediatrician, OB-GYN or Family Physician for informed medical advice about your health or the health of your baby.

## Preemie Gifts

www.perfectlypreemie.com

www.babylinq.com

www.preemiestore.com

www.earlyarrivalinc.com

## Activities In the NICU

www.miraclebebe.com

www.bevscountrycottage.com/
preemies.html

## Health & Awareness

www.preemiecare.org

www.ttmf.org

www.kristiemcnealy.com

www.preemieworld.com

## Books & Research

www.nicurollercoaster.com

www.littlemanthemovie.com

www.preemieprimer.com

www.prematurity.org

## Other Resources

_____
_____
_____
_____
_____

Made in the USA
Lexington, KY
24 January 2017